Dining with the Mayans

MY MEXICAN RECIPES COOKBOOK

Elì Arteaga
Dining with the Mayans

Table of Contents

RED ENCHILADA SAUCE 7

RED PEPPER-SOUR CREAM SAUCE 9

REFRIED BEAN BAKE 11

REFRIED BLACK BEANS 13

RICE CON QUESO 15

ROASTED TOMATO SAUCE 17

SALSA DE AGUACATE (AVOCADO SALSA) 18

SALSA DE JITOMATE COCIDA (COOKED TOMATO SAUCE) 19

SALSA SUPREMA 21

SALSA VERDE 22

SALSA XCATIC 23

SAN ANTONIO STYLE CHICKEN WINGS 24

SANTA FE SAUCE 26

SAVORY CHICKEN 28

SIZZLING STEAKS AND SALSA 31

SKINNY MEXICAN-STYLE NACHOS 33

SMALL CHICKEN FAJITAS	35
SOPAIPILLAS	37
SOPAIPILLAS 2	39
SOUTH OF THE BORDER STEW	42
SOUTHWEST BEEF FAJITAS	44
SOUTHWEST GUACAMOLE	46
SOUTHWEST RIBLETS	47
SOUTHWEST SCRAMBLED EGGS WITH JALAPENO JELLY	49
SPANISH RICE	51
SPANISH RICE 2	53
SPICY MEXICAN TORTILLA STACKS	54
SPICY NACHOS SUPREME	56
STEPHANIE'S CARNE ASADA	58
STUFFED MUSHROOMS	60
SUPER NACHOS	62
TACO CASSEROLE	64
TACO CHICKEN WINGS	65
TACO MEATBALLS	66

TACO PIE	67
TEX-MEX BEANS WITH CORNMEAL DUMPLINGS	69
TEX-MEX HASH	71
TEX-MEX RICE	72
TEX-MEX ROASTED CHICKEN	73
TEX-MEX STEAK AND TORTILLAS	75
TEX-MEX STRATA	77
TEX-MEX TORTILLA STACK	79
TEX-MEX TUNA SALAD	81
TEX-MEX WITH SPINACH BAKE	83
TEXMEX RED SNAPPER	85
THREE BEAN BAKES	88
TOMATILLO SAUCE	89
TOSTADAS DE POLLO Y FRIJOLES	91
TRADITIONAL CALABACITAS CON LECHE	92
TURKEY RANCHERO	93
ZUCCHINI RELISH	94
ZUNI VEGETABLE STEW	95

Copyright 2021 by **Elì Arteaga** All rights reserved.

In no way is it legal to reproduce, duplicate, or transmit any part of this document in either electronic means or in printed format. Recording of this publication is strictly prohibited, and any storage of this document is not allowed unless with written permission from the publisher. All rights reserved.

The information provided herein is stated to be truthful and consistent, in that any liability, in terms of inattention or otherwise, by any usage or abuse of any policies, processes, or directions contained within is the solitary and utter responsibility of the recipient reader. Under no circumstances will any legal responsibility or blame be held against the publisher for any reparation, damages, or monetary loss due to the information herein, either directly or indirectly. Respective authors own all copyrights not held by the publisher.

Legal Notice:

This book is copyright protected. This is only for personal use. You cannot amend, distribute, sell, use, quote, or paraphrase any part of the content within this book without the consent of the author or copyright owner. Legal action will be pursued if this is breached.

Disclaimer Notice:

Please note the information contained within this document is for educational and entertainment purposes only. Every attempt has been made to provide accurate, up-to-date, and reliable, complete information. No warranties of any kind are expressed or implied. Readers acknowledge that the author is not engaging in the rendering of legal, financial, medical, or professional advice.

By reading this document, the reader agrees that under no circumstances are we responsible for any losses, direct or indirect, which are incurred as a result of the use of the information contained within this document, including, but not limited to, —errors, omissions, or inaccuracies

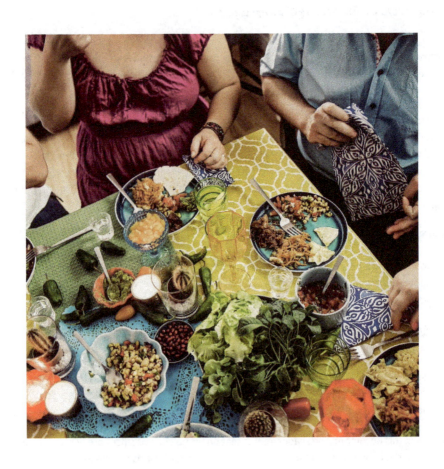

RED ENCHILADA SAUCE

Ingredients

- 10 each Large red chile pods
- 1 1/2 teaspoons Flour
- 4 each Garlic cloves
- 1/4 teaspoon Cumin
- 1 teaspoon Cilantro (optional)
- 1 1/2 teaspoons bacon drippings
- 1 each Small onion chopped
- 1 each Salt and pepper to taste
- 1 tablespoon Oregano

Directions

Boil chile pods in a small saucepan with 8-12 oz of water until soft. Place chiles, oregano, onions, garlic, and salt and pepper in a blender. Liquefy mixture.

In a 2 qt. saucepan, heat bacon drippings, and brown flour. Add the chile mixture and simmer for 30-45 minutes.

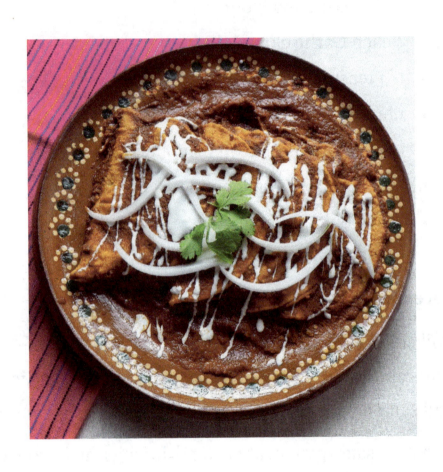

RED PEPPER-SOUR CREAM SAUCE

Ingredients

- 3 each Red Bell Peppers*
- 1 each Red Jalapeno Pepper*
- 1/2 cup Dairy Sour Cream
- 1 teaspoon Sugar

* Peppers should be roasted and peeled.

Directions

Place bell peppers and chile in a food processor work bowl fitted with a steel blade or in a blender container; cover and process until well blended. Stir in sour cream and sugar. Makes about 2 cups of sauce.

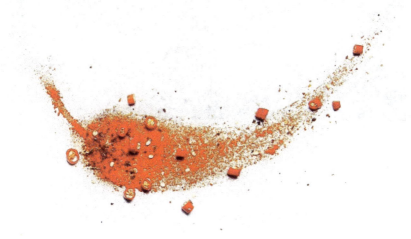

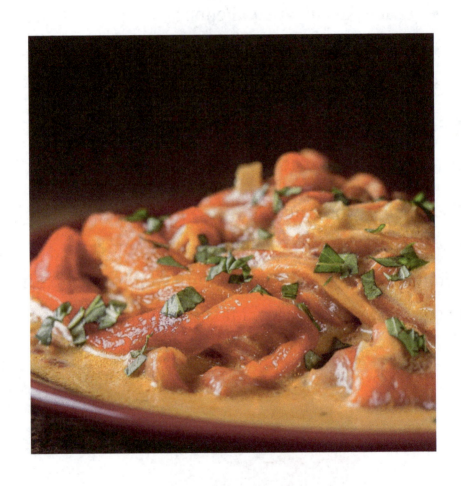

REFRIED BEAN BAKE

Ingredients

- 1 can refried beans - 16-oz
- 1 onion - finely chopped
- 1 green bell pepper - finely chopped
- 4 large eggs
- 1 1/2 cups cheddar cheese, shredded - 6-oz
- 1 teaspoon chili powder
- 1/8 teaspoon garlic powder
- 1 jar salsa - 12-oz

Directions

Mix beans, onion, green pepper, eggs, 3/4 cup of cheese, chili powder, and garlic powder. Blend well. Pour into an ungreased 9x9x2-inch pan. Sprinkle with remaining cheese. Bake, uncovered, in a 350-degree oven for about 30 minutes or until hot and firm. Heat salsa, stirring occasionally; serve with beans. Try this dish for breakfast or brunch. Serve with warmed tortillas and fresh orange slices. For brunch or supper, add some chopped green chilies (canned), sliced black olives, and maybe some marinated canned red peppers before baking. Serve with avocado slices sprinkled with lime or lemon juice and some jicama slices dipped lightly in paprika.

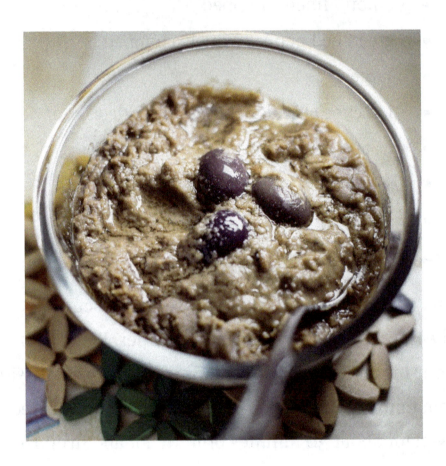

REFRIED BLACK BEANS

Ingredients

- 1/4 cup Onion; Chopped
- 2 each Jalapeno Chiles*
- 2 each Cloves Garlic - Finely Chopped
- 2 tablespoons Vegetable Oil
- 30 ounces Black Beans; Undrained - 2 Can
- 1 each Chipotle Chile*
- 1 teaspoon Red Chiles - Ground
- 1/2 teaspoon salt

* The Jalapeno peppers should be seeded with care and finely chopped.

** Chipotle Chile should be one that has been canned in Adobo Sauce, and it should be chopped.

Directions

Cook and stir the onion, jalapeno peppers, and garlic in the oil in a 10-inch skillet over medium heat until the onion is tender. Stir in the remaining ingredients and mash the beans. Cook, uncovered, occasionally stirring, until thick, about 15 minutes. Serve.

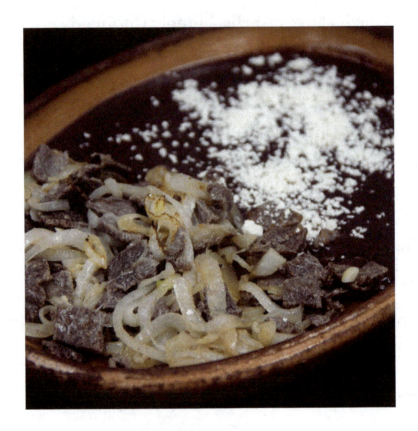

RICE CON QUESO

Ingredients

- 3 cups cooked brown rice (1 1/2 - cups uncooked), cook
- Salt and pepper
- 1 1/3 cups cooked black beans or - black-eyed peas, pint Etc. (about 1/2 cup - uncooked)
- 3 cloves garlic - minced
- 1 large Onion - chopped
- 1 small Can chiles - chopped
- 1/2-pound Ricotta cheese - thinned with little low-fat milk or Yogurt until spreadable
- 3/4-pound shredded Monterrey Jack - cheese
- 1/2 cup shredded cheddar cheese

GARNISHES (OPTIONAL):

- chopped black olives, onions, fresh parsley

Directions

Preheat oven to 350-degree F. Mix together rice, beans, garlic, onion, and chilies. In a casserole, spread alternating layers of the rice-beans mixture, ricotta cheese, and jack cheese, ending with a layer of rice and beans. Bake for 30 minutes. During the last few minutes of baking, sprinkle cheddar cheese over the top. Garnish before serving.

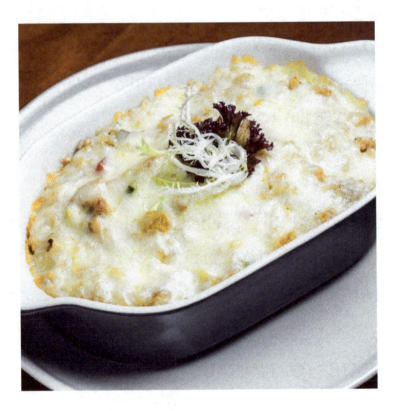

ROASTED TOMATO SAUCE

Ingredients

- 1/2 cup Onion; Chopped - 1 Medium
- 1/4 cup Carrot - Finely Chopped
- 1 tablespoon Vegetable Oil
- 2 pounds Tomatoes - Roasted & Peeled
- 1 tablespoon Basil Leaves; Fresh - Snipped
- 2 teaspoons Sugar
- 1/4 teaspoon salt
- 1/4 teaspoon Ground Red Pepper

Directions

Cook onion and carrot in oil over medium heat, occasionally stirring, until tender. Cut tomatoes into fourths; drain. Place onion, carrot, tomatoes, and remaining ingredients in food processor work bowl fitted with steel blade or in blender container; cover and process until well blended. Serve warm or cold. Makes about 3 1/2 cups of sauce.

SALSA DE AGUACATE (AVOCADO SALSA)

Ingredients

- 3 tomatillos - husks removed
- 2 cups water
- 2 large avocados - peeled and chopped
- 2 habanero chile - chopped
- 3 cloves garlic
- 1 small onion - chopped

Directions

Combine the tomatillos and water and boil until they are soft, about 10 - 12 minutes. Drain and discard the water.

Puree all the ingredients in a blender or food processor, adding a little water if needed to make the salsa smooth and creamy.

Serve with tostadas or on a bed of greens for a salad.

SALSA DE JITOMATE COCIDA (COOKED TOMATO SAUCE)

Ingredients

- 3 Medium Tomatoes - broiled
- 1/4 Onion - roughly chopped
- 1 Small Clove Garlic - peel & roughly chop
- 2 Tablespoons Peanut Oil
- 1/4 Teaspoon Salt - or to taste

Directions

To broil tomatoes:

Many Mexican recipes call for tomatoes to be roasted.

Traditionally they are put onto a hot comal and cooked until the skin is wrinkled and brown and the flesh is soft right through - this takes about 20 to 25 minutes for an 8-ounce tomato. However, since this method is very messy, it is best to line a shallow metal pan with foil and put the tomatoes in it. Place them under a hot broiler - do not have the flame too high, or the tomato will burn without cooking through - and turn them from time to time so that they cook through evenly - the skin will be blistered and charred. A medium tomato will take about 20 minutes. Blend the tomato, skin, core, and seeds into a fairly smooth sauce. The skin and core give both body and flavor to the sauce. And never mind if the skin is charred: that adds character, too. If the skin is very badly blackened and hard in places, then remove a little of it. This method of cooking tomatoes makes for a very rich-flavored sauce. Heat the oil, add the blended tomatoes and salt, and cook over a medium flame for about 8 minutes until it has thickened and is well seasoned.

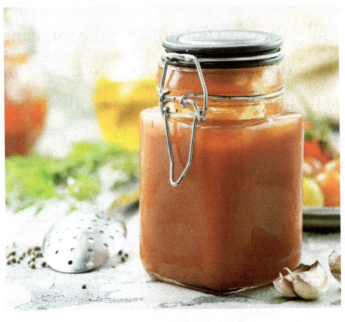

SALSA SUPREMA

Ingredients

- 1 each Large tomato - chopped
- 1 each Medium onion - chopped
- 2 each Fresh green chili - chopped
- 1 each or 4 oz can green chili
- 1/2 teaspoon Garlic salt
- 1/2 teaspoon Monosodium glutamate(option)
- Salt to taste

Directions

Combine all ingredients and chill, covered, in the refrigerator for at least one hour.

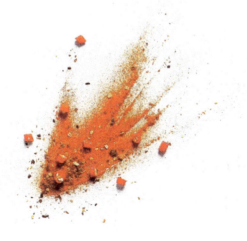

SALSA VERDE

Ingredients

- 1 can Mexican green tomatoes
- (10oz) - drained
- 1/4 cup Onions - finely chopped
- 1 tablespoon Cilantro; coarsely chopped*
- 1 teaspoon Canned Serrano chilis
- Drained, rinsed – and Finely chopped
- 1/4 teaspoon Garlic - finely chopped
- 1/2 teaspoon salt
- 1/8 teaspoon freshly ground black pepper

* Also called Chinese Parsley or Fresh Coriander.

Directions

In a small bowl, combine the tomatoes, onions, coriander, chili, garlic, salt, and pepper to taste. Mix gently but thoroughly together. Taste for seasoning.

Refrigerate if not to be used immediately. It will only keep for a couple of days. Yield: 1 cup.

SALSA XCATIC

Ingredients

- 9 xcatic chiles * - finely chopped
- 1 medium white onion - finely chopped
- 1/4 cup vegetable oil
- 1/2 teaspoon salt
- 2 tablespoons white vinegar
- freshly ground black pepper - to taste

* or substitute yellow wax hot or guero chiles.

Yucatan is identified with its native fiery chile, the Habanero, and the lesser-known chile xcatic, (pronounced sch-KA-tik). Similar to a chile guero, it is pale green, much hotter, and resembles the New Mexican chile in shape and size.

Directions

Saute the chiles and onion in the oil for 20 minutes at low heat. Place in a blender with the remaining ingredients and puree until smooth.

Serve over grilled meats, poultry, or seafood.

SAN ANTONIO STYLE CHICKEN WINGS

Ingredients

- 12 Chicken wings
- 1 cup Pace Picante sauce
- 1/3 cup Catsup
- 1/4 cup Honey
- 1/4 teaspoon Cumin - ground
- 2/3 cup Sour cream - dairy

Directions

Cut wings in half at joints; discard wing tips.

Combine 1/3 cup of the Picante sauce, catsup, honey, and cumin; pour over chicken. Place in the refrigerator; marinate for at least 1 hour, turning once. Drain chicken, reserving marinade. Place on rack of foil-lined broiler pan.

Bake at 375F. for 30 minutes. Brush chicken with reserved marinade; turn and bake, brushing generously with marinade every 10 minutes, until tender, about 30 minutes. Place 6 inches from the heat in preheated broiler; broil 2 to 3 minutes or until the sauce looks dry. Turn; broil 2 to 3 minutes or until the sauce looks dry. Spoon sour cream into a small clear glass bowl; top with remaining 2/3 cup Picante sauce. Serve with chicken.

Makes 24 appetizers. At this point, chicken may be refrigerated for up to 24 hours. To serve, place 6 inches from the heat in preheated broiler; broil for 4 to 5 minutes. Turn; broil 4 to 5 minutes or until heated through.

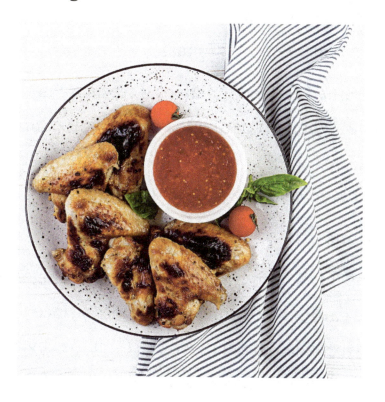

SANTA FE SAUCE

Ingredients

- 2 garlic cloves
- 1 hot chili peppers - small size
- 1 teaspoon red pepper flakes
- 3 tomatoes - * see note
- 1/2 cup chopped onions
- 1/4 cup green peppers - minced
- 4 tablespoons peanut oil
- 1/2 teaspoon salt - to taste

* Use drained canned tomatoes if fresh are not available. When preparing the hot chili, it is advised that you wear rubber gloves and be careful to avoid getting the juice of the pepper near your eyes.

Directions

Split the chiles, remove seeds, finely chop; set aside. Peel the garlic cloves and mince finely. Mince the green sweet bell pepper. Seed the tomatoes by cutting in half and gently squeeze to release some of the seeds. Chop the tomatoes into small chunks, or drain canned tomatoes thoroughly and chop.

Combine the tomatoes, garlic, chili peppers, green bell peppers, salt, and red pepper flakes in a small saucepan. Add 2 cups hot water; cover the pan and simmer for about 10-14 minutes.

Heat the oil in a heavy skillet over medium heat; add the chopped onions. Saute just until tender, about 3-4 minutes, stirring occasionally.

Place the tomato mixture into a blender and puree. Add the pureed mixture to onions in skillet. Simmer over low heat, uncovered, for about 10-12 minutes or until sauce has thickened. Make this sauce and use it for any purpose, such as over scrambled eggs, roast chicken, cheese, or chicken enchiladas.

Serving Ideas: With scrambled eggs, enchiladas, chicken, cheese souffle.

SAVORY CHICKEN

Savory Chicken is so fast and so good you will just want to stand and eat it out of the pan.

HOME SPICE BLEND: use approximately the measurements below for spices.

For the spice blend, combine cumin, cayenne pepper, thyme, garlic and onion powders, salt, and flour. Increase the spice amounts if you are cooking more than 2 1/2 pounds of chicken.

Ingredients

- 3 Or 4 half chicken breasts - boned and skinned, Cut into pieces.
- 1 tsp cumin powder
- 1/4 tsp cayenne pepper
- 1 tsp crushed thyme
- 1/2 tsp garlic powder
- 1/2 tsp onion powder
- 1/2 tsp salt
- 1 Tbs flour
- 2 Tbs butter 1 or 2 cloves garlic, chopped

- 1 or 2 jalapeno chiles, seeded, minced
- 1/2 cup to 3/4 cup light beer

Directions

This recipe doubles easily but doesn't try to saute the chicken all at once. After the chicken is skinned and boned, rub it with your home spice blend. If you get inspired, add another spice. Let the spiced chicken sit at room temperature for about 20 minutes.

Using a heavy 12-inch skillet, heat the butter and oil and add 1 cup of the chicken pieces at a time. Saute over medium heat until golden. Remove to a plate. Saute the rest of the chicken, adding more oil if necessary. When all the chicken is sauteed, drain off any excess oil. Put all the chicken pieces back in the pan, along with the chiles and garlic, and add the beer.

A great head of steam will rise up to the most wonderful aroma. Quickly now, clamp on the lid and turn the heat to low. Check every 5 minutes and turn the chicken in the reducing broth. Cook for about 15 to 18 minutes.

If the broth cooks away toward the end of the cooking, just add a tablespoon more beer. In the end, you should be left with a nice thick glaze. Push the chicken around the beer glaze, so it all gets coated. This is about the best taco meat you will ever encounter.

Since tacos are filled with other things, the recipe above will serve 4 people unless you ate too much out of the pan.

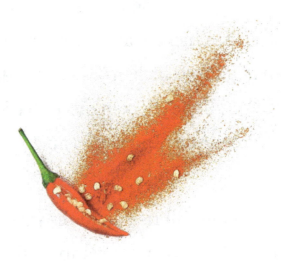

SIZZLING STEAKS AND SALSA

Ingredients

- 1-pound Boneless Beef Sirloin Steak - Cut 3/4-inch Thick
- 3/4 cup Chopped and Seeded Tomatoes
- 1/2 cup Salsa
- 2 medium Green Onions with Tops - Chopped
- 1/4 teaspoon Ground Cumin
- 1/2 cup Cheddar Cheese - Finely
- Cilantro sprigs

Directions

Combine the tomatoes, salsa, onions, and cumin and set aside. Trim the exterior fat and cut the boneless beef top sirloin steak into 4 serving-sized pieces. Place each on a flat surface, cover with waxed paper and

flatten with the bottom of a heavy saucepan, mallet, or cleaver to 1/4-inch thick. Heat a non-stick frying pan over medium-high heat for 2 minutes. Quickly pan broil the steaks for 1 minute.

Turn the steaks and top each with an equal amount of cheese. Cook 1 to 2 minutes, DO NOT overcook. Serve the steaks over the reserved salsa.

Garnish with cilantro.

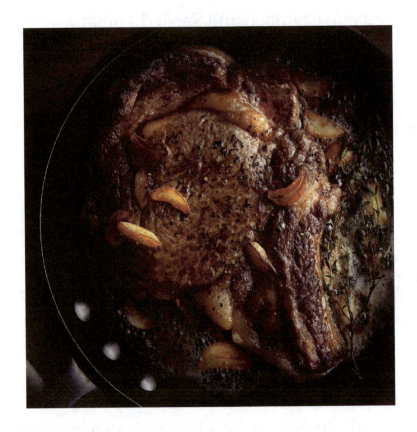

SKINNY MEXICAN-STYLE NACHOS

Ingredients

- 4 oz low-fat tortilla chips
- 3/4 can chopped onion
- 3 cloves garlic - finely chopped
- 2 tsp chili powder
- 1 jalapeno pepper - finely chopped
- 1/2 tsp ground cumin
- 1 6 oz boneless skinless chicken breast - cooked/chopped
- 1 14 1/2 oz. can Mexican-style diced tomatoes - drained
- 1 can shred reduced-fat Monterey Jack cheese - 4 oz
- 2 tbsp black olives

Directions

Preheat oven to 350 degrees. Lay chips in a 13 x 9 baking pan. Spray a large nonstick skillet with cooking spray. Heat over medium heat until hot. Add onion, pepper, garlic, chili powder, and cumin. Cook for 5 minutes

or until vegetables is tender, stirring occasionally. Stir in chicken and tomatoes. Spoon chicken-tomato mixture, cheese, and olives over chips.

Bake 5 minutes until cheese melts. Serve immediately.

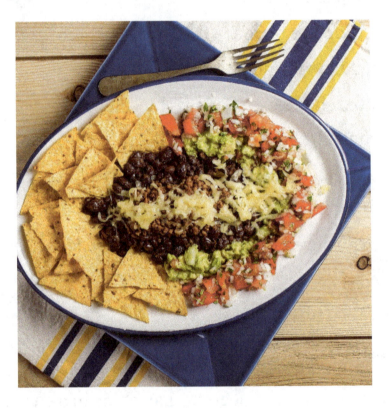

SMALL CHICKEN FAJITAS

Ingredients

- 1 pound Chicken Breast – boneless skinless

SAUCE

- 1/2 cup Soy Sauce
- 1 cup Orange Juice
- 1 tablespoon Lemon Juice
- 1 teaspoon Sugar
- 2 Cloves Garlic - crushed
- 1/2 teaspoon Ginger
- 1 tablespoon Oil
- 1 medium onion - sliced
- 1 Green pepper - sliced
- 1 Red Pepper - sliced
- 12 Flour Tortillas (6-8 inch)

Directions

Cut chicken breasts into strips 1/4" thick. Combine all sauce ingredients and pour over chicken strips. Cover and refrigerate overnight. Drain meat well and stir fry in oil along with onion and peppers until all pink color is gone from chicken pieces and vegetables are crisp-tender. Preheat sandwich maker. Trim sides from tortillas to form squares 5 X 5 or 6 X 6 inches. Brush outside of each with oil. Lay 4 tortillas on pocket grid oiled side down. Spoon chicken mixture into the triangle-shaped pockets.

Top with tortillas, oiled side up. Close lid and cook 3 minutes or until tortillas are heated through and sealed. Repeat with remaining ingredients.

Makes 12 pockets.

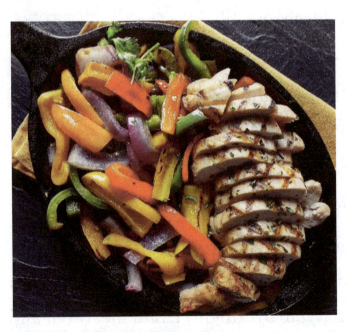

SOPAIPILLAS

Ingredients

- 4 cups Flour
- 1 tablespoon Baking powder
- 2 teaspoons Sugar
- 1 1/2 teaspoons salt
- 1/4 cup Shortening or lard
- 1 1/4 cups water or more if needed

Directions

Sift dry ingredients together. Cut in shortening until crumbly. Add water and mix until it holds together. Knead 10-15 times until dough forms a smooth ball. Cover and let sit for 20 minutes. Divide dough into two parts. Roll dough to 1/8" thickness on lightly floured board. Cut into 3" squares or triangles. Do not allow to dry; cover those waiting to fried. When ready to fry, turn upside down so that surface on the bottom while resting is on top when frying. Fry in 3" hot oil until golden brown, turning once. Add only a few at a time to maintain proper temperature. Drain on paper towels.

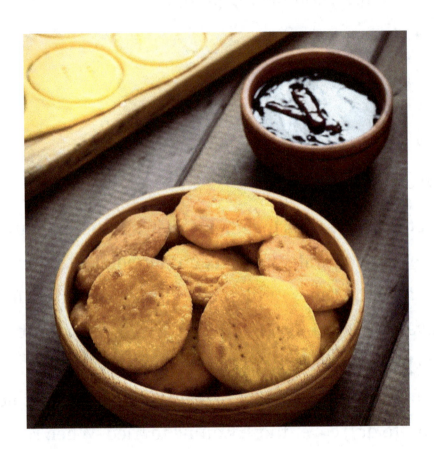

SOPAIPILLAS 2

Ingredients

- 1 package Active dry yeast
- 1/4 cup warm water (110)
- 1 1/2 cups Milk
- 3 tablespoons Lard or shortening
- 1 1/2 teaspoons salt
- 2 tablespoons Sugar
- 4 cups all-purpose flour
- 1 cup Whole wheat flour
- 1 each OIL

Directions

In a large mixing bowl, dissolve yeast in warm water. In another bowl, combine milk, lard, salt, and sugar. Heat to 110 degrees and add to dissolved yeast. Beat in 3 cups of all-purpose flour and all of the whole wheat flour. Add about 1/2 c all-purpose flour and mix until a stiff, sticky dough forms. Place dough on a floured board and knead, adding more flour as needed until dough is smooth and non-stick.

Place dough in a greased bowl turning over to grease top. Cover and let stand at room temp—1 hour. Punch dough down. The dough may be covered and chilled as long as overnight. Knead dough on a lightly floured board to expel air. Roll dough out, a portion at a time, to slightly less than 1/8" thick. Cut in 2"X 5" rectangles or 3" squares for appetizers. Place on lightly floured pans and lightly cover. If you work quickly, you can let cut sopaipillas stay at room temp up to 5 min; otherwise, refrigerate them until all are ready to fry. In a deep, wide frying pan or kettle, heat 1 1/2 - 2 inches oil to 350 on a deep-fat frying thermometer. Fry 2 or 3 at a time. When the bread begins to puff, gently push the bread into the hot oil several times to help it puff more evenly. Turn several times and cook just until pale gold on both sides, 1-2 minutes total. Drain on paper towels.

Serve immediately or place in a warm oven until all are fried. Or if made ahead, cool, cover and chill, or freeze. To reheat, bake uncovered in a 300 oven, turning once, just until warm, 5-8 min. Do not overheat, or they will become hard. Makes 2 dozen large sopaipillas or about 4 dozen small ones.

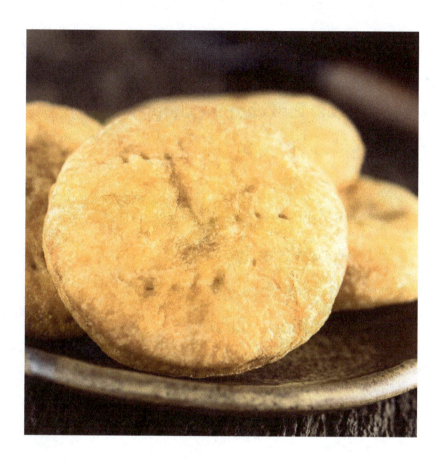

SOUTH OF THE BORDER STEW

Ingredients

- 1/4 cup butter
- 2 pounds Boneless round steak - cubed
- 5 Zucchini - sliced thin
- 3 cups Corn
- 1 can (4 oz) grin chilies - chopped
- 2 cloves garlic - minced
- 1 teaspoon salt
- 1/4 teaspoon Oregano
- 1/4 teaspoon Cumin
- 1 cup Cheddar cheese - shredded
- 1/4 cup Chopped cilantro

Directions

In a large skillet, melt butter: brown meat, a few pieces at a time.

Remove from the skillet as they brown. Saute zucchini in skillet for 7-10 minutes.

Return meat and add corn, chilies, garlic, salt, oregano, and cumin.

Simmer, occasionally stirring, for about 12-15 minutes or until meat is tender. Stir in cheese until melted. Garnish with chopped cilantro and serve.

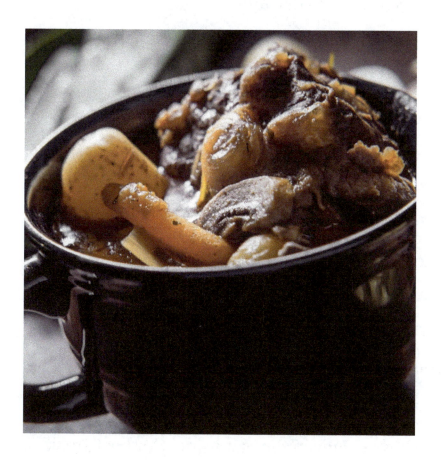

SOUTHWEST BEEF FAJITAS

Ingredients

- Cucumber Salsa
- Southwest Relish
- Southwest Guacamole
- 1 pound Top Round Steak - Boneless*
- 1/4 cup Lime Juice
- 2 tablespoons Vegetable Oil
- 2 teaspoons Red Chiles - Ground
- 2 Cloves Garlic - Chopped
- 8 Flour Tortillas**

* Round Steak should be cut about 1/2 inch thick. ** Flour Tortillas should be 10 inches in Diameter and be warmed.

Directions

Prepare Cucumber Salsa, Southwest Relish, and Southwest Guacamole; set aside. Cut beef steak diagonally across the grain into thin slices, each 2 X 1/8-inch. Mix remaining ingredients except for tortillas in a glass or plastic bowl; stir in beef until well coated. Cover and refrigerate for at least 1 hour. Set oven control to broil. Place beef slices on rack in broiler pan. Broil with tops 2 to 3 inches from heat until brown, about 5 minutes. Place 1/8 of the beef, some Cucumber Salsa, Southwest Relish, and Southwest Guacamole in the center of each tortilla. Fold one end of the tortilla up about 1 inch over the beef mixture; fold right and left sides over the folded end, overlapping fold-down the remaining end. Serve with remaining salsa, relish, and guacamole.

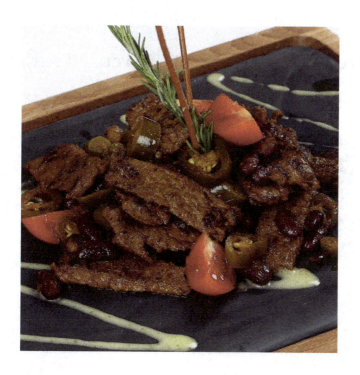

SOUTHWEST GUACAMOLE

Ingredients

- 5 each avocado; Ripe - Peel & Pit
- 4 each Cloves Garlic - Finely Chopped
- 1 cup Tomato; Chopped - 1 Medium
- 1/4 cup Lime Juice
- 1/2 teaspoon salt

Directions

Mash avocados in a medium bowl until slightly lumpy.

Stir in remaining ingredients. Cover and refrigerate for 1 hour. Makes 3 cups of dip.

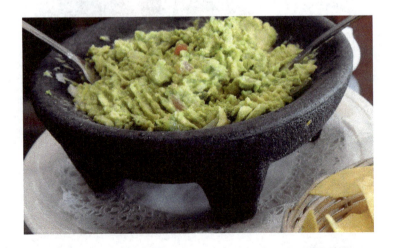

SOUTHWEST RIBLETS

Ingredients

- 1/2 cup Onion; Chopped - 1 medium
- 2 tablespoons Vegetable Oil
- 1 tablespoon Red Chiles - Ground
- 6 each Juniper Berries; Dried - Crush
- 3 each Cloves Garlic - Finely Chopped
- 1/2 teaspoon salt
- 1/2-ounce Baking Chocolate - Grated
- 1 cup Water
- 2 tablespoons Cider Vinegar
- 6 ounces Tomato Paste - 1 can.
- 2 tablespoons Sugar
- 3 pounds Pork Back Ribs; Fresh*

* Rack Of ribs should be cut lengthwise across the bones. Have the butcher do this with his meat saw.

Directions

Cook and stir onion in oil in a 2-quart saucepan for 2 minutes. Stir in ground red chiles, juniper berries, garlic, and salt.

Cover and cook for 5 minutes, stirring occasionally. Stir in chocolate until melted. Pour water, vinegar and tomato paste into a food processor work bowl fitted with a steel blade or into a blender container. Add onion mixture and sugar; cover and process until well blended. Heat oven to 375 Degrees F. Cut between pork back ribs to separate. Place in a single layer in roasting pan, pour sauce evenly over pork. Bake uncovered 30 minutes; turn pork. Bake until done, about 30 minutes longer.

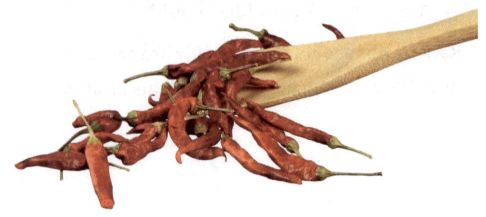

SOUTHWEST SCRAMBLED EGGS WITH JALAPENO JELLY

Ingredients

- 1/2 onion
- 3 tablespoons margarine
- 6 eggs
- 2 tablespoons jalapeno jelly
- 3 ounces cream cheese

Directions

Fit the steel knife blade into the work bowl of the food processor.

Process onion until chopped in 1/4-inch pieces. Melt margarine in a medium skillet. Saute onion in skillet until tender. With steel knife blade still attached, process eggs, jelly, and cream cheese until smooth, about 30 seconds. Pour mixture into skillet with onions and scramble until eggs are dry.

Serving Ideas: A special breakfast or brunch dish.

Notes: Serve with plenty of fresh fruit, homemade muffins, sausage or ham, and coffee.

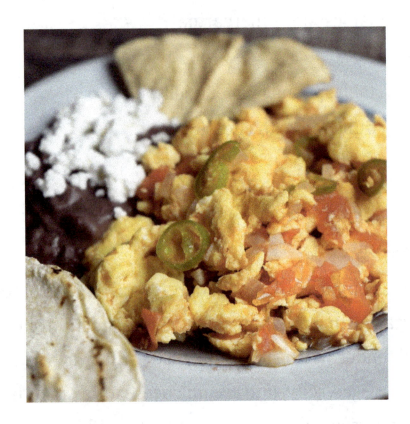

SPANISH RICE

Ingredients

- 3 tablespoons Shortening
- 1 1/2 cups Rice
- 1/2 cup Onion - sliced
- 1/2 cup Bell pepper - sliced
- 1 each 14 oz can whole tomatoes
- 1 each medium clove garlic - minced
- 1 teaspoon Black pepper
- 2 teaspoons salt
- 3 cups Water

Directions

Melt shortening in a large skillet. Add rice and brown. When rice is golden brown, reduce heat and add onion, bell pepper, tomatoes, garlic, and pepper. Mix well and add 1 1/2 cups warm water or enough to just cover the rice. Add salt. Cover and let simmer until almost dry. Add remaining water, cold, a little at a time, cooking over low heat until fluffy. Note: You may substitute peeled seeded green chili for the bell pepper.

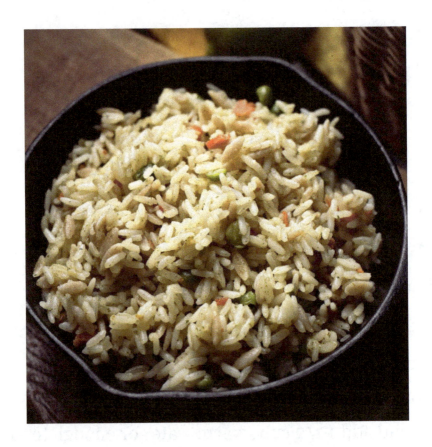

SPANISH RICE 2

Ingredients

- 1 cup uncooked long-grain rice
- 4 tablespoons Oil
- 2 tablespoons Diced bell pepper
- 3 tablespoons Diced onion
- 1 teaspoon dried parsley flakes
- 3 ounces Tomato paste
- 2 each Cloves garlic - minced
- 2 1/2 cups Coldwater
- 3/4 teaspoon salt

Directions

Lightly brown rice in oil over medium heat, stirring constantly. Add bell pepper and onion and saute' five minutes more, stirring often.

Remove from heat; add parsley, tomato paste, and garlic. Stir well, and then add water and salt. Heat mixture to boiling, cover tightly, and simmer 20 to 30 minutes or until liquid is absorbed. Remove from heat and let steam 10 minutes before serving.

SPICY MEXICAN TORTILLA STACKS

Ingredients

- 1 can Pinto Beans (15oz), drained - rinsed
- 1 can Black Beans (15oz), drained - rinsed
- 1 can Corn (16oz)
- 1 can Chopped Green Chilies (4oz)
- 1 large Onion - chopped
- 1 large Green Pepper - chopped
- 5 Flour Tortillas
- 1 cup Monterey Cheese - pre-shredded
- 1 cup Cheddar Cheese - pre-shredded
- 1 large Jar Salsa

Directions

Preheat oven 425". Combine beans and corn in a large bowl. Stir in chilies, onion, and green pepper. Lay one tortilla at the bottom of a greased two-quart souffle or casserole dish. Spoon a small amount of bean mixture over the tortilla. Top with equal amounts of Monterey Jack and cheddar cheese. Continue alternating layers of tortilla, bean mixture, and cheese mixture until you end with a cheese layer. Bake covered at 425" for 10 minutes. Serve with salsa.

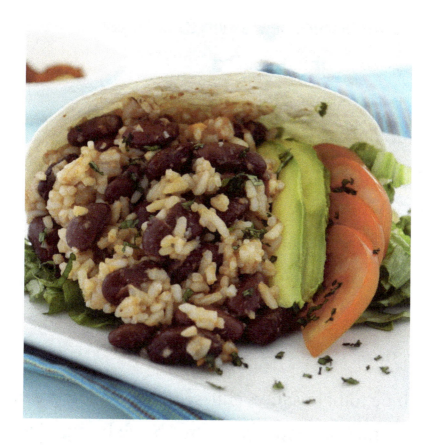

SPICY NACHOS SUPREME

Ingredients

- 8 ounces Tomato Sauce
- 4 ounces Diced Green Chiles
- 1/2 cup Chopped Green Bell Pepper
- 1 Green Onion - Sliced
- 1/4 teaspoon Hot Pepper Sauce
- 10 ounces Tortilla Chips
- 2 cups Shredded Cheddar Cheese
- 1 Avocado
- 1 teaspoon Lemon Juice
- 1/2 cup Sour Cream
- Jalapeno Slices - Optional

Directions

Combine tomato sauce, chiles, green pepper, green onion, and hot pepper sauce in a bowl; let stand for 15 minutes. Place tortilla chips in a shallow 8" X 10" baking dish. Pour sauce over chips; sprinkle grated cheese overall. Broil nachos for 3 minutes or until cheese melts. Just before serving, seed, peel, and mash avocado. Stir in lemon juice. Spoon avocado mixture and sour cream on hot nachos and top with jalapeno slices. Serve immediately.

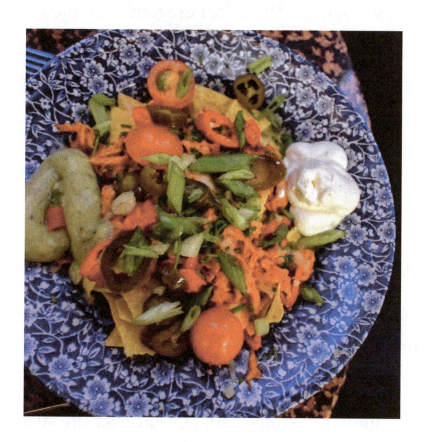

STEPHANIE'S CARNE ASADA

Ingredients

- 1 20 oz top sirloin steak
- 2 tablespoons Vegetable oil
- 1/2 teaspoon Dried leaf oregano - crushed
- 1/2 teaspoon salt
- 1/4 teaspoon Coarsely ground pepper
- 1/4 cup Orange juice
- 1 tablespoon Lime juice
- 2 teaspoons Cider vinegar
- 2 Orange slices - 1/2" thick

Directions

Place steak in a shallow glass baking dish. Rub with oil on each side.

Sprinkle with oregano, salt, and pepper. Sprinkle orange juice, lime juice, and vinegar over the steak. Cover and refrigerate overnight for best flavor or several hours, turning occasionally.

To cook, bring meat to room temperature. Prepare and preheat charcoal grill (or gas grill). Drain meat, reserving marinade. Place steak on the grill. Top with orange slices. Occasionally spoon reserved marinade over steaks as they cook. Grill 3-4 minutes on each side, or until medium-rare. Cook longer if desired. Remove orange slices to turn steak. Replace orange slices on top of the steak.

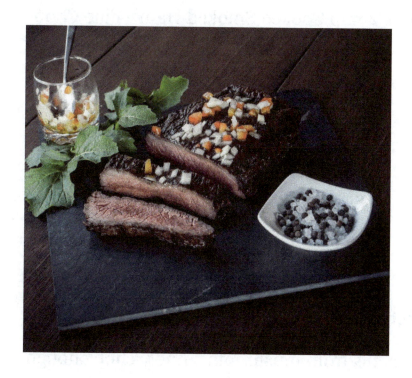

STUFFED MUSHROOMS

Ingredients

- 24 each Mushroom - Medium
- 2 tablespoons Margarine or Butter
- 1/4 cup Onion; Chopped - 1 Medium
- 2 tablespoons White Wine - Dry
- 1/4 cup Breadcrumbs - Dry
- 1/4 cup Cooked Smoked Ham - Fine Chop
- 2 tablespoons Parsley - Snipped
- 1 tablespoon Lime Juice
- 1 each Clove Garlic - Finely Chopped
- 1 teaspoon Oregano Leaves - Dried
- Dash of Pepper
- 1/2 cup Cheese; Finely Shredded*

* Use Monterey Jack Cheese in this recipe.

Directions

Cut stems from mushrooms; finely chop enough stems to measure 1/4 cup. Heat margarine in a 10-inch skillet just until bubbly. Place mushroom caps, topsides down, in margarine. Cook uncovered until mushrooms are light brown; remove mushrooms with a slotted spoon. Cook and stir onion in the same skillet until tender; stir in wine. Simmer uncovered 2 minutes. Mix in chopped mushroom stems and remaining ingredients except for cheese and mushroom caps; cool slightly. Shape mixture into 24 small balls; place 1 in each mushroom cap. Sprinkle with cheese. Set oven control to broil. Place mushroom caps on rack in broiler pan. Broil with tops 3 to 4 inches from heat until cheese is melted, about 3 minutes.

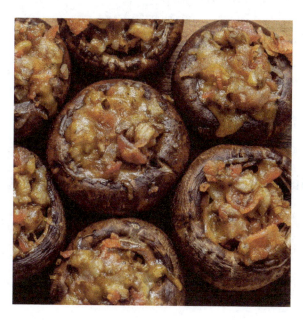

SUPER NACHOS

Ingredients

- 1 can refried beans
- 1 can green chilis
- 2 cups Monterey jack cheese
- 2 cups cheddar cheese - (Velveeta best)
- 3/4 cup taco sauce
- 1/2 cup sliced black olives - or to taste
- 1 tsp lemon juice
- 1 cup sour cream
- tortilla or nacho chips

Directions

Brown ground beef, add onion, and cook until tender. Drain fat, add salt and pepper to taste. Spread refried beans in a 10"x13" baking dish. Top with meat. Place green chilis on top. Mix Monterey jack and cheddar cheese together and sprinkle on top. Drizzle taco sauce over evenly and bake uncovered 20-25 minutes 400 degrees. Remove from oven. Mix black olive with lemon juice and spread them on top. Cover with sour cream and serve at once with chips.

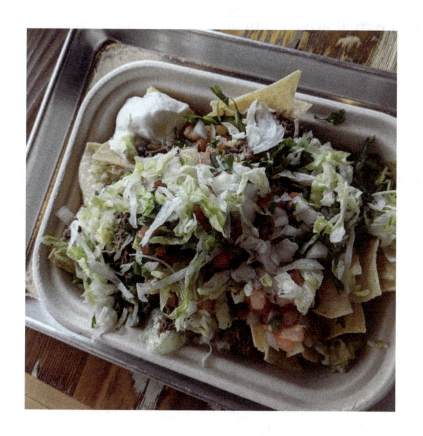

TACO CASSEROLE

Ingredients

- 1 pound Hamburger
- 1 Envelope taco seasoning mix
- 1 can Tomato sauce
- 1 1/2 cups Water
- 1 cup Grated cheese (more if you - want it)
- bag baked tortilla chips

Directions

Saute meat in skillet. Add taco seasoning mix, tomato sauce, and water.

Bring to a boil, reduce heat, and simmer uncovered 15 min. Add tortilla chips; mix, being careful not to break the chips. Pour into a 2-inch-deep by 8 inches round or square baking dish. Bake in the oven to 400 F 10-15 minutes. Top with cheese.

TACO CHICKEN WINGS

Ingredients

- 2 1/2 pounds Chicken Wings
- 1 Envelope Taco Seasoning Mix*
- 2 cups Dry Breadcrumbs
- 1 Jar (16oz) Taco Sauce **

* 1-1/4 oz Old El Paso ** Old El Paso

Directions

Remove wing tips and discard. Cut wings at joint. Combine breadcrumbs and taco seasoning mix; mix well.

Preheat oven to 375. Dip each chicken piece in taco sauce, then roll in breadcrumbs, coat thoroughly. Place on a lightly greased baking sheet. Bake for 30-35 mins.

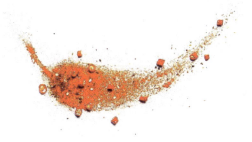

TACO MEATBALLS

Ingredients

- 1 pound Beef - ground
- 1 cup Green pepper
- 1 cup Rice - cooked
- 2 teaspoons Garlic salt
- 11 ounces Cheddar cheese soup
- 1 cup Onion
- 1 cup Celery
- 2 each Egg - beaten
- 8 ounces Taco sauce

Directions

Mix all but the last two ingredients. (I puree vegetables in a blender rather than chopping.) Form meatballs and place in 2- 1/2 qt. dish.

Bake at 350 degrees for 30 minutes. While baking, heat taco sauce and soup on the stove. Pour over meatballs and bake for another 30 minutes.

TACO PIE

Ingredients

- 1 package Crescent rolls
- 1 package Taco mix
- 2 cups Corn chips - crushed
- 1 cup Cheddar - shredded
- 1 pound Hamburger
- 1/2 cup Water
- 1 cup Sour cream

Directions

Cook hamburger, taco mix, and water according to package directions.

Place unrolled crescent dough in an ungreased pie plate to form crust.

Sprinkle with half of the corn chips and top with hamburger mixture.

Spread sour cream on top and cover with cheese and remaining chips.

Bake at 375 degrees for 20 minutes or until heated through.

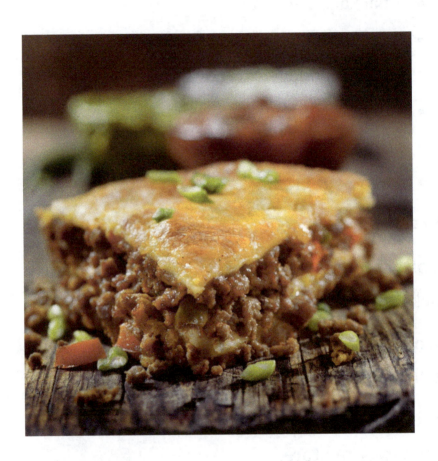

TEX-MEX BEANS WITH CORNMEAL DUMPLINGS

Ingredients

- 1/3 cup Flour
- 1 teaspoon Baking powder
- Beaten Egg White
- 2 tablespoons Cooking Oil
- 1 cup Chopped Onion
- 15 ounces Can Garbanzo Beans - drained
- 15 ounces Can Tomato Sauce
- 2 teaspoons Chili powder
- 1 1/2 teaspoons Corn-starch
- 1/3 cup Yellow Cornmeal
- 1/4 teaspoon salt
- 1/4 cup Skim Milk
- 3/4 cup Water
- Clove Garlic - minced
- 15 ounces can Red Kidney Beans - drained
- 4 ounces Can diced green chili pepper
- 1/4 teaspoon salt

Directions

In a med mixing bowl, stir together flour, cornmeal, baking powder, and 1/4 t salt; set aside. In a small bowl, combine egg white, milk, and oil; set aside.

In a 10" skillet, combine the water, onion, and garlic. Bring to boiling; reduce heat. Cover and simmer for 5 minutes or till tender. Stir in garbanzo beans, kidney beans, tomato sauce, drained green chili peppers, chili powder, and 1/4 t salt.

In a small bowl, stir together cornstarch and 1 T water. Stir into bean mixture. Cook and stir till slightly thickened and bubbly. Reduce heat.

For dumplings, add milk mixture to cornmeal mixture; stir just until combined. Drop dumpling mixture from a Tablespoon to make 5 mounds atop bean mixture.

Cover and simmer for 10-12 minutes or till a toothpick inserted in the center of a dumpling comes out clean.

TEX-MEX HASH

Ingredients

- 1 pound Ground beef
- 1 each Green pepper - chopped
- 1/2 cup Rice - uncooked
- 2 teaspoons salt
- 3 each Onion - sliced
- 1 can Tomato - whole (medium can)
- 1 teaspoon Chili powder
- Pepper - dash

Directions

Preheat oven to 350 degrees. Pan fry ground beef until light brown in skillet. Drain fat. Add onions & peppers and cook until onion is tender. Stir in the rest of the ingredients and heat until warm. Pour in a casserole dish, cover, bake for 1 hour.

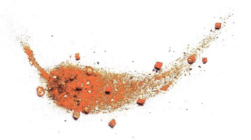

TEX-MEX RICE

Ingredients

- 3/4 cup Onion - chopped
- 2 tablespoons Olive Oil
- 1 cup Rice - raw
- 1/4 teaspoon Black Pepper
- 2 Garlic Cloves
- 2 1/2 cups Vegetable Broth
- 1 1/2 teaspoons Ground Cumin
- 1 Red Bell Pepper

Directions

Mince garlic. Remove seeds and dice bell pepper.

In a dutch oven, cook onion, garlic, and raw rice in oil until onion is tender and rice is lightly browned.

Add chicken broth and bring to a boil. Stir in cumin and black pepper.

Cover tightly and simmer for 20 minutes. Remove from heat. Stir in bell pepper. Let stand covered until all liquid is absorbed, about 5 minutes.

TEX-MEX ROASTED CHICKEN

Ingredients

- 1 teaspoon ground cumin
- 1 teaspoon chili powder
- 1/2 teaspoon Basil
- 1/4 teaspoon salt
- 1 tablespoon white wine vinegar
- 1 (3 Lb.) broiler-skinned
- 2 cups coarsely chopped zucchini
- 1 1/4 cups unpeeled - seeded & coarsely chopped tomatoes.

Directions

Combine the first 6 ingredients; stir well & set aside.

Remove giblets & neck from chicken & discard. Rinse chicken & pat dry. Rub outside of the chicken with spice mixture. Place chicken, breast side down in a deep 3 qt. Casserole. Cover with wax paper & microwave at high 8 to 9 min. Turn chicken, breast side up & microwave covered with wax paper at high 8 to 9 min.

Remove chicken to serving platter. Reserve drippings in casserole. Let chicken stand covered 15 min. Add vegetables to drippings; toss to coat. Microwave at high 3 to 4 min. Or until crisp-tender, stirring halfway through the cooking process. Arrange vegetables around chicken.

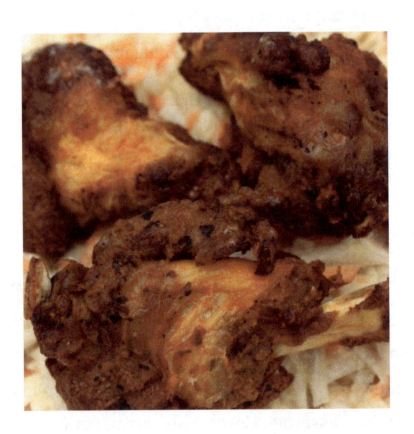

TEX-MEX STEAK AND TORTILLAS

Ingredients

- 1 1/2 pounds Boneless sirloin each about thick
- 1/2 cup Corn oil
- 3 teaspoons Garlic - chopped
- 4 tablespoons Red wine vinegar
- 1-pound Ripe tomatoes
- 1/2 cup Onion - chopped fine
- 1/4 cup Red chilies - chopped fine
- 1/4 cup Coriander - chopped fine
- 12 Flour tortillas

Directions

Prepare a very hot charcoal fire.

There should be about 6 individual steaks. Cut each of these in half. Blend the oil, 2 tsp garlic, and 3 tbsp vinegar in a flat dish. Add the steaks, turning to coat the pieces well. Set aside.

Core the tomatoes but do not peel them. Cut them into 1/4-in. cubes and put them in a mixing bowl. Add the onion, chilies, coriander, remaining garlic, and vinegar. Blend well. Set this sauce aside.

Put about 4 slices of steak at a time on the hot grill and cook for 1 min. or less to a side, depending on the desired degree of doneness. Simultaneously, add a similar number of tortillas and cook them for a few sec. to a side just to heat through. Do not heat for long, or they will dry out.

Place one piece of steak in the center of a warm tortilla, spoon a little sauce over the meat and fold the side of the tortilla over the ends up to enclose the meat. Eat like a sandwich.

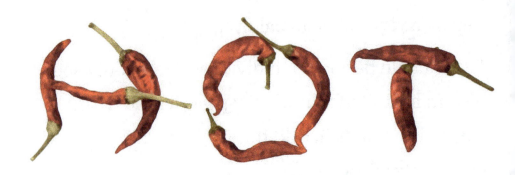

TEX-MEX STRATA

Ingredients

- 1/2-pound Hot Italian sausage
- 6 ounces Red peppers; roasted – drain and chopped
- 6 ounces Green peppers - fried
- 6 Firm white bread - quartered
- 1 1/2 cups Monterey Jack cheese
- 1 1/2 cups Milk
- 1 teaspoon Chili powder
- 1/2 teaspoon salt
- 6 Eggs - beaten

Directions

In a medium skillet, saute sausage for 10 minutes or until lightly browned. Cool slightly; cut crosswise into thin slices. Place in bowl. Add peppers; toss to combine. Preheat oven to 350~. Generously grease 2 qt. shallow baking dish. Reserve 6 bread quarters; place remainder in prepared dish. Sprinkle with cheese and the sausage mixture; arrange reserved bread on top.

Set aside. In a medium bowl, beat eggs with milk, chili powder, and salt until mixed; pour over bread in the dish.

Bake for 1 hour or until the center is set. Let stand 10 minutes before serving. Makes 6 servings.

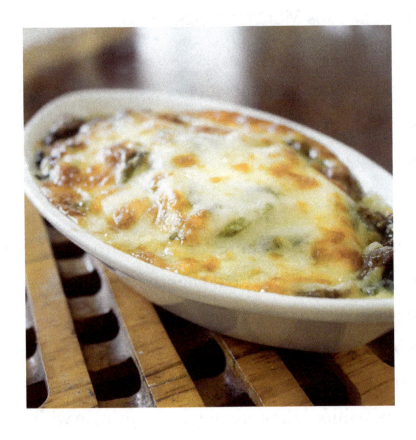

TEX-MEX TORTILLA STACK

Ingredients

- 1 9-oz. pkg. (2 cups) frozen
- Chopped cooked chicken
- 1 cup Finely chopped – peeled Jicama
- 1/2 cup Taco sauce
- 8 10-inch flour tortillas
- 1 6-oz. container frozen
- Avocado dip - thawed
- 2 cups Chopped lettuce
- 1 16-oz. can refried beans With green chili peppers or Mexican-style beans – drained And mashed
- 1 8-oz. carton reduced-fat or Regular dairy sour cream
- 1/2 cup Chopped red sweet pepper
- 1/3 cup Sliced green onion
- 1 cup Shredded lower-fat or Regular cheddar cheese – or Monterey Jack cheese with
- Jalapeno peppers

- 1/4 cup Sliced pitted ripe olives
- Taco sauce (optional)

Directions

THAW CHICKEN: In a medium mixing bowl, combine chicken, jicama, and the 1/2 cup taco sauce; set aside.

Place one of the flour tortillas on a platter. Spread with half of the

chicken mixture. Spread half of the avocado dip onto a second tortilla; place, avocado side up, atop chicken. Sprinkle with half of the lettuce. Top with a third tortilla; spread with half of the beans. Top with another tortilla; add half each of the sour cream, red pepper, green onion, and cheese.

Repeat layers, ending with remaining sour cream, red pepper, green onion, and cheese. Sprinkle with olives. Serve right away or cover and chill for up to 3 hours.

To serve, cut into wedges. Pass taco sauce.

Makes 8 main-dish servings.

TEX-MEX TUNA SALAD

Ingredients

- 2 cans of solid white tuna in water - drained and flaked.
- 1/2 cup sliced ripe olives
- 1/2 cup Sliced green onions w/tops
- 1/2 cup thinly sliced celery
- 2/3 cup Pace Picante Sauce
- 1/2 cup Dairy sour cream
- 1 teaspoon ground cumin
- Lettuce leaves – or Shredded lettuce
- 12 Taco shells – or 3 cups Tortilla chips

Directions

Combine tuna, olives, green onions, and celery in a medium bowl. Combine Pace Picante Sauce, sour cream, and cumin; mix well. Pour over tuna mixture; toss lightly. To serve, line taco shells with lettuce leaves; spoon tuna mixture into shells. Or, line individual serving plates with shredded lettuce, top with tuna mixture, and surround with tortilla chips.

Drizzle with additional Pace Picante Sauce; top with additional sour cream, if desired.

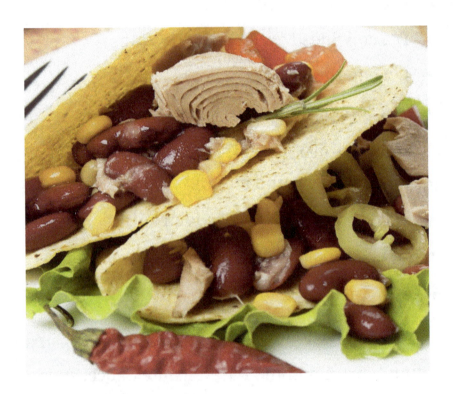

TEX-MEX WITH SPINACH BAKE

Ingredients

- 2 cups Bisquick baking mix
- 1/2 cup Water - cold
- 1 pound Ground beef
- 1 package taco seasoning mix
- 1 cup Water
- 10 ounces Spinach*
- 1 cup Cheese - ricotta
- 1/3 cup Green onions - chopped
- 1 1/2 cups Cheddar cheese - shredded
- 1 cup Sour cream
- 1 egg - lightly beaten

* frozen, thawed, chopped, and squeezed dry.

Directions

Heat oven to 350~F. Combine baking mix and 1/2 c cold water; stir until soft dough forms.

Press dough into the bottom of greased 13x9" baking dish.

Cook ground beef in a large non-stick skillet until brown. Stir in taco seasoning mix (dry) and 1 c water.

Bring to a boil; reduce heat and simmer 15 minutes, stirring occasionally.

Spoon mixture over dough.

Combine spinach, ricotta cheese, and onions; spread over ground beef mixture. Combine Cheddar cheese, sour cream, and egg, spoon evenly over spinach mixture. Bake 30 minutes or until set. Let stand 5 minutes before serving.

TEXMEX RED SNAPPER

Ingredients

- 2 tablespoons olive or salad oil
- 1 Large onion - chopped
- 2 cloves garlic - minced
- 4 teaspoons Sugar
- 1 teaspoon salt
- 1/4 teaspoon Cinnamon - ground
- 1/4 teaspoon Cloves - ground
- 5 cups Peeled, seeded - chopped tomato
- 1 1/2 teaspoons Each: water & lemon juice
- 1 tablespoon Cornstarch
- 2 Jalapenos, seeded - chopped
- 2 tablespoons capers
- 5 1/2 pounds Red Snapper, cleaned, scaled Head removed
- 1/3 cup Pimento stuffed green olives Sliced thin.
- 3 tablespoons chopped fresh cilantro

Directions

Heat oil in a wide frying pan over med heat; add onion and garlic and cook, often stirring, until onion is soft. Stir in sugar, salt, cinnamon, cloves, and tomatoes. Cook, stirring, over high heat until a thick sauce form (abt. 8 min.).

Blend together lemon juice, water, and corn-starch; stir into tomato mixture. Cook until mixture boils and turns clear; remove from heat. Stir in chiles and capers. Rinse fish, pat dry. Place a 24-inch sheet of foil crosswise in a large roasting pan. Grease foil lightly (spray with Pam), then place fish on foil; pour hot tomato sauce over fish. Bake, uncovered, in a 400 F. oven until fish flakes when prodded with a fork in the thickest part (abt. 45 min). Baste frequently with sauce during the last 15 min. of baking.

Skim watery juices off the sauce with a spoon, then stir the sauce to blend.

Lift foil, fish, and clinging sauce and slide onto a platter; drizzle with remaining sauce in the pan. Garnish with olives and cilantro.

To serve, cut fish to the bone, then lift off each serving.

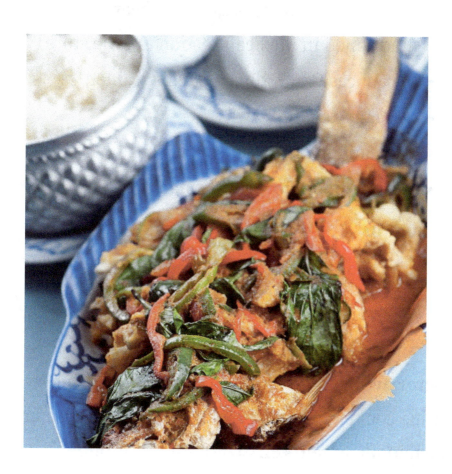

THREE BEAN BAKES

Ingredients

- 16 ounces Can Great Northern Beans – undrained 16 ounces can Chili beans – undrained in Mexican section - of the store)
- 16 ounces Can Kidney Beans - drained
- 1/3 cup Ketchup
- 1/3 cup Firmly packed brown sugar
- 1/2 teaspoon Powdered ginger

Directions

In a 2-quart microwave-safe casserole or dish, combine all ingredients. Mix well. Cover with Waxed Paper.

Microwave on HIGH for 8 - 11 minutes, stirring twice during cooking. If thicker juice is wanted, Micro in two min increments on 80% power. Stir often.

CROCKPOT Directions. Combine all ingredients, mix well. Cover - cook on High setting for 2 hours. If thicker juice is wanted, remove the cover, cook 1 hour longer, stirring occasionally.

TOMATILLO SAUCE

Ingredients

- 1/4 cup red onion - chopped
- 1/4 cup fresh cilantro - snipped
- 1/4 teaspoon salt
- 1/2-pound tomatillos - cut into halves
- 2 each serrano chiles - canned*

* Use 2 canned serrano chiles, rinsed and seeded, or 1 fresh serrano chile, seeded.

Directions

Place all ingredients in food processor work bowl fitted with steel blade or in blender container, cover, and process until well blended. Makes about 1 1/4 cups of sauce.

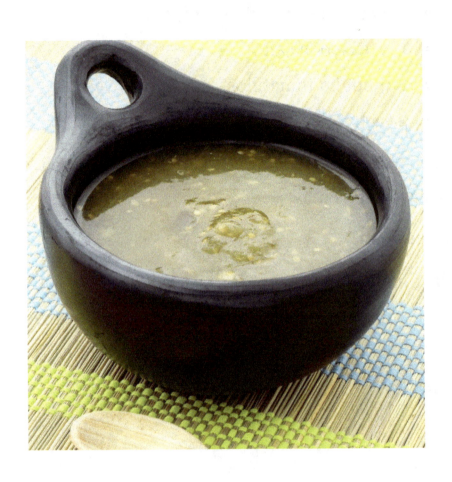

TOSTADAS DE POLLO Y FRIJOLES

Ingredients

- 2 tortillas
- 2 cups cooked - mashed black beans (or refried beans)
- 2 cups chicken - shredded
- 1 tomato - wedged
- 1 cup string beans - cook & cool
- 1 head lettuce - shredded
- 1 green bell pepper - sliced
- 2 green onions - diced
- 1 can plain green olives - chopped
- 1 cup Cheddar cheese - grated
- 2 tablespoons Hot sauce

Directions

Lay a tortilla on each plate; spread with a layer of beans. Lay chicken on beans. Toss together vegetables and cheese; and mound on top of chicken. Sprinkle hot sauce on top.

TRADITIONAL CALABACITAS CON LECHE

Ingredients

- 4 each medium summer squash - sliced
- 1/4 cup butter or margarine
- 1 each 15 oz can corn - drained
- 1/2 cup onion - thinly sliced
- 1/2 teaspoon salt
- 1 each dash pepper
- 1 each 4 oz can chopped green chili
- 1 cup milk
- 1/2 cup grated cheddar cheese

Directions

Saute' squash in butter until soft. Reduce heat and add corn, onions, salt, pepper, and green chili. Mix well and add milk. Simmer until well blended. Add cheese and cover until cheese is melted.

TURKEY RANCHERO

Ingredients

- 4 Turkey thighs
- 1 package Enchilada sauce mix
- 6 ounces Tomato paste
- 1/4 cup Water
- 4 ounces Monterey Jack - grated
- 1/3 cup Lowfat yogurt or sour cream
- 1/4 cup Green onions - sliced
- 1 1/2 cups Corn chips - crushed

Directions

With a sharp knife, cut each thigh in half; remove bone and skin. Place in crockpot. Combine enchilada sauce mix with tomato paste and water. The mixture will be thick. Spread on thighs. Cover; cook on LOW for 7 to 8 hours or until tender. Turn pot on HIGH. Add cheese; stir until melted. Spoon into an au gratin dish or shallow casserole. Spoon yogurt over turkey. Sprinkle with onions. Top with corn chips.

ZUCCHINI RELISH

Ingredients

- 2 cups Zucchini - Shredded
- 1/4 cup Fresh Cilantro - Snipped
- 2 tablespoons Lime Juice
- 2 tablespoons Vegetable Or Olive Oil
- 1 teaspoon salt
- 1/4 teaspoon Sugar
- 1/4 teaspoon Pepper

Directions

Mix all ingredients in a glass or plastic bowl. Cover and refrigerate for at least 1 hour. Makes about 1 1/4 cups of relish.

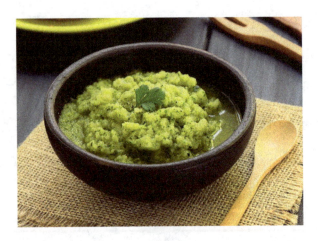

ZUNI VEGETABLE STEW

Ingredients

- 3/4 cup onion - chopped
- 1 each clove garlic - finely chopped
- 2 tablespoons vegetable oil
- 1 each red bell pepper; large*
- 2 each chile; medium size**
- 1 each jalapeno chile - seed & chop
- 1 cup squash - cubed***
- 29 ounces chicken broth - 2 cans
- 1/2 teaspoon salt
- 1/2 teaspoon pepper
- 1/2 teaspoon coriander - ground
- 1 cup zucchini - thinly sliced
- 1 cup yellow squash - thinly sliced
- 17 ounces whole kernel corn - drained
- 16 ounces pinto beans; drained - 1 can

* Bell pepper should be seeded and cut into 2 X 1/4-inch strips. ** Chiles should be either poblano or

Anaheim and should be seeded ***Use either Hubbard or acorn squash. (about 1/2 pound)

Directions

Cook and stir onion and garlic in oil in a 4-quart Dutch oven over medium heat until onion is tender. Stir in bell pepper, poblano and jalapeno chiles. Cook for 15 minutes. Stir in Hubbard squash, broth, salt, pepper, and coriander. Heat to boiling; reduce heat. Cover and simmer until squash is tender, about 15 minutes. Stir in the remaining ingredients. Cook uncovered, occasionally stirring, until zucchini is tender, about 10 minutes.

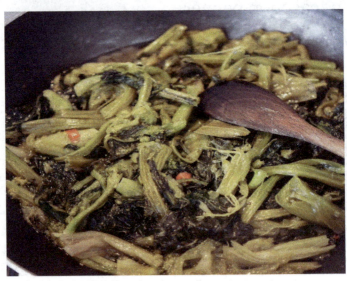

CPSIA information can be obtained
at www.ICGtesting.com
Printed in the USA
LVHW080755090621
689684LV00012B/1517